A Plan for a Single-Payer Health Care System

A Plan for a Single-Payer Health Care System

✦

The Best Health Care in the World

Charles H. Chen, MD, FACOG

iUniverse, Inc.
New York Bloomington Shanghai

A Plan for a Single-Payer Health Care System
The Best Health Care in the World

iUniverse books may be ordered through booksellers or by contacting:

iUniverse
1663 Liberty Drive
Bloomington, IN 47403
www.iuniverse.com
1-800-Authors (1-800-288-4677)

ISBN: 978-0-595-47158-4 (pbk)
ISBN: 978-0-595-71112-3 (cloth)
ISBN: 978-0-595-91438-8 (ebk)

Printed in the United States of America

Contents

Preface

The health care system in the United States is in crisis and needs to be reformed right now. In order to clarify the complex health care system, I will explain the scope of the health care system and give the definitions of *single-payer system, multi-payer system,* and *universal health care system.*

The scope of the health care system includes coverage, funding, and management. Health insurance should cover every citizen. Fees paid for health care costs should be funded through various methods. Management of the system includes collecting all the funds, paying out all health care costs, monitoring the costs and quality of care, contracting and setting up policy for all health care participants, collecting and reporting health care outcome data, educating consumers on health issues and disease prevention, estimating the health care budget, and improving the system.

A *single-payer system* is one in which health insurance covers every citizen. The central or federal government acts as one entity to collect all the funds through a general taxation for citizens who pay income tax (parents have to pay for their children), to collect the money from the states for those citizens whose income is below the state poverty level, and to sell low-cost insurance to those citizens who do not pay income tax or to uninsured citizens. The government needs to pass a law that requires every citizen to carry health insurance; this is the same as universal health care. However, one payer (the federal government) will manage the system. A single-payer system is not socialized medicine, nor is it government bureaucracy. It is not free care; it is cost-saving and more efficient health care management.

A *multi-payer system* is one in which health insurance does not cover citizens who cannot afford to buy insurance or do not want to buy insurance. The current U.S. health care system is a multi-payer system. Funding is through private insurers, individuals, programs such as Medicare and Medicaid, health maintenance organizations (HMOs), and employers. A multi-payer system creates multiple managers, so the administrative costs are very high and the quality of health care is difficult to evaluate. Multiple managers create serious problems for health care management.

A *universal health care system* is one in which every citizen is required to have health insurance coverage. Funding is similar to a multi-payer system, but the government passes a law mandating that private insurance companies sell affordably priced policies to uninsured citizens. As with a multi-payer system, there are multiple managers (in multi-payer mode). Universal health care (in multi-payer mode) emphasizes universal health *coverage*, but it does not have a well-designed health care *management* plan.

The health care system is so complex that no single person has the experience and knowledge to handle every aspect of it. However, my experience and research have given me the background to be able to address what types of reform are important. In my private practice, as a doctor specializing in obstetrics and gynecology, I have been dealing with the health care system for twenty-nine years. This book is based on the knowledge I have obtained from my own experience and research; from talking to insurance carriers about medical claims; from chairing departments that deal with hospital administration; from discussing the health care system with my colleagues, including doctors, nurses, and other medical professionals; from attending lectures sponsored by hospitals, pharmaceutical companies, and business schools; and from reading health care journals containing discussions of domestic and foreign health care issues.

Before I entered medical school and became a medical doctor, I went to visit my uncle's clinic in Taiwan in 1967 and 1968. I observed his busy medical practice. At that time, patients respected doctors. The consumer (the patient) had to pay cash. The total fee included an examination or consultation and drugs from his clinic. Patients were very happy, and they were aware of their financial responsibility. If a patient did not have the money, he or she would borrow it from relatives or friends in order to pay the doctor. It was his or her responsibility to pay back the money that he or she had borrowed. However, sometimes my uncle would see a patient without charge if he was aware that the patient was unable to pay the fee. In more than one case, I saw a patient's tears running down his cheeks in appreciation of the doctor's kindness.

This basic unity between consumer and provider persists up to today. Modern-day medical practice has become a business of financial arrangement, but ordinary citizens cannot do anything about the health care industry's focus on profit. Few citizens even understand how their health care plans work.

I have reviewed the international health care systems and then summed up the best health care system in this book. However, each country has to modify its strategy according to its own people's likes and needs. Based on my research, I have concluded that a single-payer system is the best system for the United States.

After comparing all the health plans in the United States, I have found that the Medicare plan (the U.S. government-sponsored universal health care plan for people over sixty-five years) is the best health care plan (Urban Institute 2003). Medicare is a single-payer system. Another example is the Veterans Administration health care system, which is also a single-payer system. "It provides excellent quality care," said Reinhardt (2004). In a peer-reviewed paper published in the *Annals of Internal Medicine*, research done by the RAND Corporation showed that the quality of care received by patients of the Veterans Administration scored significantly higher overall than did comparable metrics for patients in the rest of the U.S. health care system.

When I reviewed foreign health care systems, Taiwan National Health Insurance (NHI) consistently received a 70 percent public-satisfaction rate (Lu and Hsiao 2003). NHI is an example of universal health care funded by general taxation—a single-payer system. Most citizens pay a general tax and enroll in NHI; citizens who do not pay income tax can purchase low-cost NHI insurance plans. They pay the same rate as the citizens who pay the general tax rate. The administrative cost is about 2 percent of the NHI total expenditure (Lu and Hsiao 2003). This translates into huge savings for consumers. Their total health spending, as a percentage of the gross domestic product (GDP) was about 6 percent versus the United States' 13 percent (OECD; and Lu and Hsiao 2002).

Currently, the United States' health care expenditures amount to about 16 percent of the GDP (Davis et al. 2007). Taiwan NHI had tried universal health care funded by a multi-payer system, but it had failed. The United Kingdom's National Health Service (NHS) is another example of universal health care funded by general taxation. Their total health spending was about 7.8 percent of their GDP versus the United States' 15.2 percent (OECD 2006). The legislators have the authority to remove the NHS director very quickly if the citizens' satisfaction is below a certain level.

Introduction

Health is a basic human right. However, our current health care system fails to ensure that everyone has access to the assistance he or she needs. The public needs to support a government system that is not run as a profit-seeking business.

The medical and health care business is unique and should operate differently from other business models. The following provides an overview of the problems in the health care system and some solutions for them.

Free-market economists think of the health care system as being like the production of cars; if there is competition among many car manufacturers, then consumers can get a better car at a lower price. But this theory cannot apply to a health care system. Because there are many variables, consumers cannot evaluate and compare the costs and outcomes of quality care. Economists also think that consumers can get free medical care from a single-payer system; therefore, consumers may abuse the system and medical costs will be too high to control. However, most people do not want to undergo unnecessary medical procedures or take unnecessary medications. Therefore, in a single-payer system, most patients who visit a doctor would probably do so because they truly felt they needed assistance, not because it was free. A well-designed and well-conceived health care system will prevent consumers and providers from abusing the system. In fact, the corporate giants—insurance carriers, pharmaceutical companies, and hospital executives—can take advantage of the current free-market system; they are the ones who abuse the health care system.

Free-market economists also think health insurance companies can get the best price from a hospital because there are many hospitals to compete for their business. In reality, the health insurance company has no alternative but to sign a contract with a particular hospital because most of the insurance company's subscribers are not willing to drive too far from their homes for the treatment of most common diseases, which account for a majority of hospitalizations. The hospital has overhead-expense data, which it uses to support its demands that the insurance carrier reimburse for more expenses each year, despite negotiations and bidding. Many hospitals, whether for profit or not for profit, always want to have more money than they can generate.

Furthermore, health insurance companies cannot lose money; if they predict they are going to have a deficit next year, they will raise insurance premiums. The salary of a CEO of an insurance company is huge, regardless of whether the CEO does the morally right thing or the morally wrong thing. A free market can create this kind of unfair business, in which someone can receive such a salary without adequately representing and satisfying consumers.

On the other hand, there are many doctors; therefore, an insurance company can reduce its payment to doctors, and the doctors cannot afford to refuse the contract because there is so much competition. Still, there are some greedy doctors as well. They try to cheat the system, but it has nothing to do with funding the system, as free-market economists believe. Under a free-market health care system, it is only the consumers and honest providers who do not get any benefit at all. All others in the industry receive huge benefits.

Well-designed systems, making use of modern advances in information technology, can monitor the behaviors of consumers and health care providers very closely. Individual health care records can be monitored using computers. This would help to prevent abuse of the system. The honest behavior of doctors and patients should prevail in the practice of medicine. Preauthorization, managed health care, a consumer-controlled system, and the like will not work if an individual doctor or patient intends to act dishonestly. The immoral behavior of consumers and doctors is learned, not innate. Therefore, education and setting up policy play an important role in preventing abuse. The policy must be disclosed to all the health care participants.

Not the inflow of money into the health care system, but the management of the system—controlling the cost of health care and monitoring quality of care and care outcomes—is the key problem with the current system. There are too many middlemen to manage the system in the United States now. The United States spends almost 16 percent of its GDP on health care, the highest percentage in the whole world, yet not all U.S. citizens have health care coverage. Health care outcomes are near the bottom of all industrialized countries (8th Annual Tamkin Symposium 2006).

A value-based health care system (Porter 2006) will have tremendous impact for cost-saving and high-quality care. It will create a center of excellence that will monitor health care costs and compare them with the quality of care and health care outcomes.

A single director will be responsible for the design and management of the entire health care system. Although assistants will also be necessary, the director should be very hands-on. It is important that the director is compensated well. The health care system's design is the utmost important process in order to carry out a successful health care system. The success or failure of a country's health care system will depend on a thoughtful, sophisticated, and well-designed system; here I will call it the *National Health Care System* (NHCS). The National Health Care System I refer to is a single-payer system with general taxation, administered and managed by central government.

There are many so-called experts in each sector of the health care system. The medical economist, the professor of a business school, the health insurance company promoter, the hospital administrator, the medical society, the health care provider, the government agent, and the consumer all proclaim that they know and can solve the problems in the current system. It is like the parable "The Blind Men and the Elephant," in which one man touches the large elephant's side, then says the elephant is a big wall; another touches the elephant's ear, then he says the elephant is a fan, and so on. It is difficult to find the one person who understands all of the issues affecting the health care system.

1

Essential Concepts of the Health Care Business

There are two important concepts behind a successful health care business plan: cooperation and making the right choices.

Payers and all other health care participants should cooperate with each other to carry out quality care at low cost. The manager (in a single-payer system) will contain the administrative costs and make the right choices for all health care participants. Just as the Department of Defense designs a strategy to defend the entire country and is not subject to free-market competition, the health care system should operate as a single unit to care for the nation's citizens. The free market in the current health care system has not worked as expected (it was supposed to contain costs and provide high-quality care), and health care expenditures continue to soar. Health is a basic human right. It should be a higher priority than national defense. While it is necessary for participants in the health care industry to make a profit, it is immoral to take advantage of human suffering in an effort to make large sums of money. Before designing an effective system, several factors must be considered.

Consumers and Providers (Medical Doctors)

The most important element in any health care system is the knowledge that all of the business originates from consumers and providers. All other health care–related participants are secondary. Doctors should have autonomy to treat patients. However, because doctors would be paid with taxpayer money in a single-payer system, their contracts should be monitored carefully. I discuss this further in chapter five. Consumers should also have restrictions on the use of the health care system, as I outline in chapter four. The NHCS will act as the financial manager and care advisor for all providers and consumers.

Medical Economics

Free-market economic theory cannot apply to a health care system. In a single-payer system, under certain situations in particular areas of health care, health care providers can still apply free-market theory in order to give better quality care at a lower cost. Providers can compete, using efficiency and smart business operation, in order to gain a higher profit margin. They can create a center of excellence and attract more patients.

Consumers and providers (medical doctors) need to understand the basic concept of medical economics. Education for both consumers and providers (medical doctors) from NHCS should emphasize the medical cost as a direct result of the actions of providers and consumers. There will be no middleman to take advantage of doctors' and patients' business, except the government. This is a huge advantage for both doctors and patients.

Funding Models

A universal health care system (in multi-payer mode) is funded through private insurance, self-payment, employers' insurance, Medicare, HMO, or state/county assistance programs. Under this system, it is required that every citizen has health insurance. Congress needs to pass a law that requires every citizen to have health insurance. However, because payers are multiple in a universal health care system, there are many managers (middlemen) to manage the system. Universal health care funded by a multi-payer system is doomed to fail. For example, during Mr. Bill Clinton's presidency, health care reform that proposed a universal health care system was attempted. However, it was funded by multiple payers, so there would have been multiple managers. The system not only had high administrative costs, but it also had serious problems regarding health care management.

A single-payer system is one in which the central or federal government collects all the funds through general taxation of citizens who pay income tax. The government sells low-cost, affordable health insurance to citizens who do not pay income tax or to uninsured citizens. For citizens whose income is below state poverty level, the state is required to pay for their insurance. As with universal health care, Congress needs to pass the law that requires every citizen to have health insurance. Because there is one payer, there is only one manager of the system.

A multi-payer system is funded similarly to universal health care, except there are uninsured members of the population who cannot afford to buy health insurance or do not want to. Because there are many payers, there are many managers (middlemen). This is the current U.S. health care system.

Private Health Insurance

The government should allow private health insurance carriers to operate and sell health insurance plans to wealthy consumers or to any citizen who does not like the single-payer system. However, private insurance and government-run health insurance should be independent; they should not cover each other as primary or secondary insurances. Private insurance should pay for all the health care costs. Government insurance cannot and should not cover the coinsurance as a secondary insurance, and vice versa. If government insurance (single-payer system) makes a payment as the primary, and private insurance makes a payment as the secondary, it will create a relay responsibility of payment. This is analogous to a rich person who buys and owns two cars, one for regular driving and one for luxury enjoyment. However, he or she cannot drive both cars at the same time.

I emphasize that every citizen has to pay the general health care tax, even if he or she does not use the governmental health insurance. At some point in their lifetimes, most citizens will find the need for the governmental insurance. For example, they will have such governmental health care coverage in case they cannot afford to pay for their private insurance. Consumers who have both can switch insurances at any time of the year.

Additionally, private insurers must sell their plans to consumers who have preexisting conditions. Because a consumer already has the government insurance as a backup, he or she will be able to switch to the government insurance plan if a private insurance will not sell them a plan that covers preexisting diseases. In order to compete with lucrative businesses, private insurance companies will have to offer their plan to any consumer, regardless of preexisting conditions.

Private insurers should consider that it is a common misconception that all preexisting conditions will use more services. Some preexisting conditions never recur. Assuming that specific preexisting conditions can recur and may need more services, insurance carriers can design a plan customized to a consumer's needs. For example, they will sell an option for a private bed or a first-class bed when the patient is admitted to the hospital. Private insurers should also consider cost. An office visit to a doctor is not very expensive. The only expensive charges come from the hospital, from surgery in the hospital, from the laboratory, and from imaging services. In order to have a higher profit margin, private insurers must negotiate prices for those services. They should pay 100 percent of those charges and should not charge coinsurance to the consumers.

Single-Payer System

This system needs to have a very sophisticated and well-designed management plan to do a good job. The government becomes the middleman between providers and consumers, responsible for the financial management of the system. Information technology is now advanced enough to be used to track all health care expenses and outcomes.

In the suggested single-payer system, NHCS will give a contract to only those health care participants who pass the standard performance criteria. NHCS will set up the criteria and a value-based result scoring system (Porter 2006). Every citizen should receive a printout of the policy and understand the policy completely. If every citizen understands the principle behind this system, all citizens will support the government in these policies.

2

National Health Care System Design

Each country's central government should establish a department such as the National Health Care System (NHCS). NHCS is a government-sponsored single-payer health care system, paid for with a general tax (refer to the description of a single-payer system in the preface).

Director of NHCS

The director has more responsibility to all of the country's citizens than the secretary of the defense department. The head of the country should appoint the director of NHCS and have this appointment confirmed by Congress. The director should be reappointed every two to four years, and citizens should give yearly feedback regarding their level of satisfaction. From the results of the citizens' feedback, the director of NHCS can be removed quickly, particularly if the satisfaction rate is below a certain level.

Every provider should have a provider identification number in order to carry out the NHCS program more efficiently. Currently in the United States, every health care provider has a national provider identifier (NPI). Every citizen should have a health care card issued by NHCS, similar to a Social Security card. This will enable NHCS to carry out the program smoothly.

The director of NHCS should be a medical doctor who practices medicine and has clinical experience. If this person also has business experience, it will be a bonus for NHCS. The director should know what is going on in health care practice. Health care is not a hypothetical or theoretical business. If the director does not have business experience, he or she will quickly learn the necessary skills pertaining to secondary or tertiary health care business participants. If a director is from outside the medical field (a businessperson), it will be more difficult to learn practical medicine and to know what is going on in the medical field. Additionally, the director should be a medical professional because the NHCS director will represent the interests of both the consumers and the providers of health care. The director of NHCS should be well compensated, due to the complexities and demands of the job.

Division Directors

The NHCS director needs the following division directors:

- Director of the information technology division—will program all health care participants' networks and their databases.

- Director of the provider division—will set up and enforce the provider contract policy.

- Director of the consumer division—will set up and enforce the consumer policy.

- Director of the hospital division—will set up and enforce the hospital contract policy.

- Director of the laboratory division—will set up and enforce the laboratory contract policy.

- Director of the imaging services division—will set up and enforce the imaging center contract policy.

- Director of the special medical clinic division—will set up and enforce the special clinic contract policy.

- Director of the specialized surgical center division—will set up and enforce the specialized surgical center contract policy.

NHCS Policy Setup

The director of NHCS and the division directors form the department of the NHCS. In addition to the responsibilities listed above, the department will set up the policy regarding value-based data collection and reportable results of health care participants' performance. NHCS criteria need to be reviewed and changed as medical practice changes. Patient and doctor satisfaction will make the system work, and their dissatisfaction will cause it to fail. Therefore, a great amount of preliminary research, performed by NHCS, is necessary to address the needs of both groups. In order to contain health care costs, every country has to pay attention to these two factors. Not because the government wants to restrict service to patients or reduce payments to doctors, but for all citizens' satisfaction.

It is vitally important to explain the policy to consumers and health care providers before NHCS issues health care insurance cards to consumers and signs the contract with health care providers. It is my observation that not all citizens are paying much attention to their own health issues, nor do they research current health issues. There will be a certain percentage of people who will want to take advantage of the system. To prevent this, the detection and prevention of fraudulent claims is extremely important. The government must announce this clearly when NHCS commences. NHCS should set up toll-free telephone lines for people to call in and report possible fraud, or consumers and providers can report possible fraud through e-mail.

Consumer Education of Health Issues—Preventive Medicine

NHCS should spend a certain percentage of its budget on health education for all citizens. This is essential. Healthy citizens will save billions of dollars in future medical costs. It will cost more to treat diseases as they arise than to provide preventive education and care. NHCS should request an accredited college in each specialty to submit their written materials on preventive care, then NHCS should assemble the information and create the final texts. NHCS should then post that preventive medicine information on its Web site or distribute a booklet containing the information to each cardholder when he or she applies for the health care card. Because most citizens have a computer at home, consumers will be able to download the information. This should include all of the important screening and yearly checkup schedules. Consumers can set up their own schedules and reminders on their computers, which will translate into NHCS savings on expenditures.

3

The Director of a National Health Care System

The NHCS Director and Eight Division Directors

The director of NHCS will select eight division directors, listed in chapter two, to form the departmental members. The division director must visit or interview participants monthly, face-to-face, to acquire feedback from them in the first two years of operation. The NHCS director and division directors should also have a monthly meeting to improve the system as time goes by. As NHCS grows, the director will need to learn and improve the system constantly.

Health Care Expenditures Report

At the end of a fiscal year, the NHCS director will need to report the health care expenditures in relationship to the GDP. These reports should be posted on the NHCS Web site, or mailed to each health care participant.

This seems like trivial extra work for NHCS, but it is imperative to let every citizen know these numbers, so that every citizen will pay attention to the issue, which indirectly affects the containment of medical wastes and costs. If the citizens do not pay attention, medical costs will increase, and so will their health care taxes.

Performance Measurement

NHCS should set the standard criteria for health care providers' performance scores. There are three different aspects of care for which data should be collected and measured: economic, provider (doctor) performance, and consumer feedback.

From an economic standpoint, high-quality care should be provided at a low cost. Health care providers belonging to these sectors include hospitals, special medical clinics (refer to chapter four for definition), laboratory services, outpatient imaging centers, specialized surgical centers (refer to chapter ten for definition), and medical devices and equipment.

In the United States, there is a Department of Health and Human Services, the Agency for Healthcare Research and Quality (AHRQ), the Centers for Medicare and Medicaid Services (CMS), the National Quality Forum (NQF), and the National Quality Measures Clearinghouse (NQMC). They are responsible for quality of care and health care outcomes measurement. The NHCS director can and should integrate those existing agencies into one under NHCS, because one agency can process and collect the data uniformly and more efficiently.

Doctors' performance plays a major role in health care service. However, setting up the performance criteria is very difficult for a private practitioner. The NHCS director should consult with an accredited college in each specialty to set up the performance criteria; for example, continuing medical education and practice behavior. NHCS should integrate those criteria into the providers' contract policy requirement (refer to chapter five).

Patients should be allowed to rate the performance of their health care providers via a feedback mechanism; NHCS can do this by posting questionnaires on its Web site. Consumers are the recipients of their health care outcomes. The data collection is easy to carry out. This consumer point of view will have some influence on the health care providers' practice behaviors, and the providers will be more careful to perform their duties. However, these may not be accurate measurements of a health care provider's performance because they are subjective evaluations.

Recently in the United States, there has been a trend to promote pay for performance (P4P) for medical doctors. Unfortunately, current pay-for-performance criteria are for processes only; they are not direct measurements of high-quality medical care at a low cost (for a detailed explanation, refer to the section "Fee Schedule," below). The current criteria may cost more to operate, and care of lesser quality may result. Until the criteria are appropriately set up by each specialty college's consensus, it will not be a good idea to carry out a pay-for-performance system. But it may apply to the health care participants in such sectors: hospital, outpatient laboratory service, outpatient imaging service, special medical clinic, specialized surgical center, and obstetric delivery center.

The director of NHCS should consider all three measurements and then integrate these into the scoring systems.

Health Care Card

The health care card should have two components: a consumer's personal data, similar to a Social Security card, and a link to the consumer's personal electronic medical records. NHCS should keep the electronic medical record of each cardholder in a centralized office.

Health care providers can retrieve a patient's electronic medical record via the Internet each time a patient comes for a visit. This can save a lot of overhead at the doctor's office. Each time a consumer goes to see the doctor or to the hospital, the doctor or hospital will retrieve that cardholder's electronic medical record and subsequently enter all new records. All other services, such as laboratory tests and imaging reports, will enter this consumer's electronic medical record too. Therefore, each time this consumer goes to see a doctor or to a hospital in any location, his or her medical record will be there. This not only saves time, but also can reduce medical error due to a miscommunication or incomplete medical information. The doctor's office paper chart should be obsolete.

When issuing the health care card to the consumer, it is mandatory to include policy instructions. Consumers will need to pass a written examination on policy in order to get a card. Patients under certain conditions, such as newborns, people who cannot read or write, people with severe mental retardation, and the like, will be exempt from the examination. The director of NHCS should write the test. The contents should include what the NHCS goals are, what each division's function is, questions about preventive medicine, questions about personal responsibility for health issues, and so on. The test can be taken online or at a local branch of NHCS.

When selling a health care card to uninsured consumers, NHCS will hire an expert to figure out the price. It will be the same price or less than the price for those people who pay the health care tax. Pricing will depend upon age; a ten-year card will be cheaper than a one-year card, in terms of a yearly rate.

Network of Health Care Participants

NHCS should design a computer software program that connects all of the health care participants in one network. This will save many billions of dollars in administrative costs. This can save billions of dollars in health care providers' overhead expenses too. This networking software program should be supplied to all health care participants, free of charge, in order to carry out the program with uniformity, consistency, and efficiency.

Fee Schedule

The following issues need to be considered:

(1). Fees paid to the providers per procedure code (CPT) should be the same, regardless of geographic area. This will encourage doctors to go to medically underserved or rural areas to practice medicine. Doctors who practice in rural or underserved areas get a relatively higher payment. This is the right thing to do for the country as a whole. Geographically, practicing doctors will be more evenly distributed among the states.

(2). Pay-for-Performance (P4P) for medical doctors, in theory, seems like a good idea; good performance will get more reimbursement. The problem is a question of how to define good performance and how to set up the criteria. P4P can be a micromanaged care delivery process. In the United States, there has recently been a trend to promote P4P. Current criteria for performance, written by insurance providers or government agencies, is a process of health care delivery (pre-established targets for delivery of health care services). However, although it may cost more to process, it may not improve quality of care. Human beings are not robots; the diagnosis and treatment of each person varies, dependent on many factors such as age, sex, lifestyle, and the degree of severity of illness. It is very difficult to have a fixed formula to get the result of quality performance. Doctors are required to spend many years in school and training because the diagnosis and treatment of diseases need to be customized; it is not a fixed formula.

To improve quality of care and control costs, the individual practitioner must be up-to-date on the latest medical knowledge and refine his or her surgical skill for surgical procedures. No alternative can replace individual achievement. For more information on how to attain those goals, please refer to chapter five.

Good health care providers should be rewarded with an increase in the number of patients they have. The contract-for-performance method is a more appropriate and more objective measurement than P4P. Contract for performance means the health care providers will get a contract with NHCS if they pass the performance standard. The NHCS will set up the criteria for this. (Please refer to my three measurements of performances earlier in the chapter.) If health care participants pass the standard performance score, they get a contract. NHCS should encourage the participants who pass the basic standard score to advance to a higher level of performance. Health care providers will receive more financial reward if they have more consumers; this is where NHCS comes into play. NHCS will encourage customers to choose the health care participants who have higher performance scores by publishing the participants' scores on its Web site. Most consumers will select higher-scoring providers; this encourages health care providers to compete against each other in terms of quality of care.

(3). Co-payment and coinsurance should apply to both the single-payer system and to private health insurance. The main purpose of this is to deter consumers' overutilization of services. A co-payment (or registration fee) is the payment for doctor's office visits, emergency room visits, and urgent care visits only. NHCS should use the methodology of trial and error and adjust the co-payments accordingly every year. The adjustment will depend upon the outcome of health care expenditures. Co-payments will increase if consumers overutilize services and decrease if consumers underutilize services.

Coinsurance is the money that patients must pay to providers (doctors, emergency room services, urgent care centers, and hospitals) after services are rendered and insurance has made payment. For example, if the payers (private or government) pay 80 percent, then patients pay the remaining 20 percent of the allowed charge (*allowed charge* is the reasonable charge that the government or private insurance sets up in the fee schedule). In a single-payer system, coinsurance (10 percent or 20 percent of allowable charge) should apply to doctors' office visits, emergency room visits, and urgent care visits only. If patients are required to pay a 10 or 20 percent coinsurance out of their own pocket, they will be more prudent and careful in their use of health care services. This will control overutilization of the services. The consumers will check out the treatment options and look for a doctor with a high performance score. It is similar to people when they are buying high-priced merchandise; they will be more careful to decide if they need that merchandise, and if they decide it is necessary, they will select the highest quality.

In the United States, hospitals, surgical centers, laboratories, and imaging services bill itemized charges that are unbelievably high. Consumers cannot figure out what those charges are for. A governmental single-payer (NHCS) or a private health insurance should pay 100 percent of the claims for those providers.

Annual Meeting

The NHCS director will set up the date of the annual meeting with all health care participants. At the end of the fiscal year, the director will meet with all health care participants (representatives for doctors, consumers, hospitals, laboratories, imaging services, and medical-equipment suppliers). The director will report the surplus or deficit of the health care budget. If the NHCS health care budget has a surplus, then the reimbursement rate will increase in the future. All health care participants should work together in order to achieve the goal of high-quality care at low costs.

4

Consumer Policy Setup

In order to prevent some consumers from abusing the system, the consumer policy should be disclosed to every citizen in advance when he or she receives an NHCS health card. The language and sentences of this policy need to be very concise and brief.

Medical Expense Setup

If the medical expenses from a consumer's doctor's office visits, emergency room visits, and urgent care visits reach a total of, for example, three thousand dollars (each country must decide on an upper limit for medical expenses), then the report will be sent to the medical-expense examiner, who is an NHCS employee. It should be similar to the operation of a credit card. Consumers can use up to the given credit line. If consumers' expenses are over the given credit line, there must be something wrong. A credit card company must investigate what is happening.

The medical-expense examiner should look into the report and examine the patient's record. Then the medical examiner will decide if that patient is a chronic-disease patient who needs to go to a special medical clinic (refer to definition below). Alternatively, the primary-care doctor will decide and certify, once the final diagnosis is made, that the patient should be classified as having a chronic disease and the primary-care physician will assign the patient to a special medical clinic. The followings entities belong to the category of chronic diseases: diabetes, stroke (recovery from acute stage), chronic mental disorders (dementia, Alzheimer's disease, etc.), chronic heart diseases, chronic pulmonary diseases, cancer (medical treatment after surgery and radiation), chronic kidney disease (for dialysis), rheumatologic disease, HIV, and "bad lifestyle" diseases (chronic alcoholism, smoking, and obesity).

Once patients enroll in a special medical clinic for chronic-disease care, their medical expenses are recorded as zero in their card's record because the special medical clinic will pay for them. The clinic will get paid by NHCS at a wholesale contract rate (similar to an HMO). The exact payment will depend on negotiations between NHCS and the special medical clinic.

Special Medical Clinic

A special medical clinic is a total health care delivery clinic. It should not be used for treatment of acute diseases. The clinic needs to set up the following programs for treatment of chronic diseases:

(1) Patient education

(2) Medical treatment

(3) Rehabilitation

(4) Follow-up and monitoring

(5) Collection and reporting of treatment results

Co-Payment Fee Schedule

The co-payment is the registration fee that patients pay at the time of service. The following fees are my suggestions only; they can be adjusted after trial and error: For a doctor's office visit, the co-payment should be twenty-five dollars for a primary-care physician and fifty dollars for a specialty physician. For an urgent care center, the co-payment should be fifty dollars. For an emergency room visit, the co-payment should be seventy-five dollars.

The co-payment fee schedule should adjust every year, depending on the expenditure outcomes. The fees may increase if health expenditures and overutilization of health services are high, or the fees may decrease if health expenditures are low. The reason for a high co-payment is to prevent and discourage patients' overutilization of health care services and abuse of the system.

If a patient does not agree to this arrangement, then that patient should buy private insurance or pay cash to the doctor; therefore, medical expenses on his or her NHCS health care card will show zero expenses. If a patient decides to use the NHCS card later, his or her NHCS card will start all over again. Private insurance and the NHCS insurance should be entirely independent.

NHCS should set up a Web site for patients to view their medical expenses. The Web site should also include health education articles and other materials for consumers to learn about health issues. NHCS should emphasize the importance of preventive medicine, whether it involves paying primary-care physicians to do preventive medicine or spending a certain percentage of the NHCS budget to create programs designed by an accredited college in each specialty that inform patients of important health issues, including preventive medicine. NHCS should set up a toll-free telephone number for patients to call and find such information if they do not have a computer.

Coinsurance Fee Schedule

Coinsurance is the fee patients pay to the health care providers after services are rendered and the insurance company (NHCS or private insurance) informs patients of their responsibility. This is dependent on the setup of the insurance policy. In general, it is about 10 to 20 percent of the service's allowed charge. The insurance company should show the consumer how much he or she owes providers in an explanation-of-benefits letter after services are rendered.

Coinsurance should apply only to doctor's office visits, emergency room visits, and urgent care visits. The coinsurance fee should not apply to the claims charged by hospitals, outpatient surgery centers, laboratory services, or imaging services. The charges for those services are unbelievably high and consumers cannot determine where they come from, even with an itemized list. Because doctors order those services, patients have no way to control them. Insurance companies (NHCS or private insurance) should know how to determine a reasonable price for those services, but not the patients. For that reason, 100 percent of such charges should be paid by the insurance company.

Web Site Setup

NHCS should set up a Web site for consumers to leave their feedback and comments. The NHCS network software will then be able to read and generate a summary and report of the data. Those reports will be given to the NHCS director for review. He or she will use the information to make any changes in policy for further improvement.

5

Provider (Medical Doctor) Contracts

The provider is the key player in a medical care system. In order to avoid certain bad or incompetent doctors, the following policy should be disclosed to all doctors when they sign the contract agreement.

Continuing Medical Education

Continuing medical education (CME) is essential for doctors' self-improvement. This will help a practitioner practice high-quality care at a low cost.

NHCS should establish two educational programs that will directly affect practitioner behavior. Practitioners should be given medical-economic education and should be required to attend patients' case-management meetings.

Most practitioners never learn medical economics. NHCS should hire experts to create this educational program. Practitioners should have the option of learning this via computer programs or through attending lectures in the hospital setting. However, to carry out this program in a much easier and more practical way, I recommend using the Internet and computer programs. Every practitioner would read the texts and take a test. The CME credits will be automatically recorded in each practitioner's personal-profile database.

Doctors should also be required to attend patients' case-management meetings in the facility where he or she practices (hospital, clinic, surgical center, etc.). The meeting should be held once a week or every other week, and it should cover all patients who have been treated in that facility. One member of the meeting should be a doctor, preferably a professor or comparable expert in that profession, invited from a teaching institute to give his or her comments. This educational meeting will have a direct effect on practitioner behavior. Practitioners will not only learn from their own patients' cases, but also from other doctors' cases. The person in charge of registration at the meeting will give a CME credit to the doctor who attends the meeting for the entire time. Part-time attendance in the meeting will not count for credit.

NHCS will set up the minimum credit hours for the above continuing medical education. It is easy to collect each practitioner's data in an online, networked database similar to the consumers' records.

Monitoring Practitioner Behavior

Here is an example of how advances in information technology can help to monitor practitioner behavior. If a patient has uterine myoma (fibroid of the uterus), the practitioner can order an ultrasound to see what size and how many fibroids are in the patient's uterus. If the practitioner wants to order a computed tomography (CT) scan, or magnetic resonance imaging (MRI), then the computer will show a yellow alert and ask the practitioner why he or she wants to order an MRI or a CT scan; the practitioner can then enter the reasons, and the computer will show a yellow alert again. This time it will state that a CT scan or an MRI cannot make a diagnosis of cancer and ask if the practitioner still wants to order a CT scan or an MRI. There are two options that this practitioner will have: he or she can call a radiologist and ask his or her opinion, or the practitioner can continue to order the MRI or CT scan. If the practitioner still wants to order the scan, then the computer will show the sentence "Please enter the final diagnosis." He or she can ignore the prompt to enter the final diagnosis, or he or she can enter the final diagnosis, which will turn out to be just fibroids. Both answers will be entered in this practitioner's database. The data collected from this practitioner will show a bad score because the doctor has ordered unnecessary tests (NHCS will set up the score criteria), and then NHCS will decide if it should discontinue its contract with this practitioner.

If NHCS will not contract with a practitioner, a practitioner can continue practicing medicine for privately insured patients. He or she may apply for a contract with NHCS again after updating his or her knowledge and taking a training course.

Medical Charge Card

NHCS should issue a medical charge card, similar to a credit card, to every citizen who has health insurance with NHCS. NHCS should supply a card-reading machine or software program free of charge to every contracting provider. This will greatly enhance uniformity in processing transactions. Additionally, mass production of the machines or software will cost less. It will also save providers money on overhead expenses. If a doctor's office can reduce its overhead, its net income will increase. This means NHCS can reduce the reimbursement rate, which translates into huge savings for NHCS.

Each time a patient enters the provider's office and the doctor sees the patient, a receptionist will slide the card with the time in. After the doctor finishes the examination and before the patient leaves the doctor's office, the receptionist will print out a charge slip. All data will be programmed by NHCS, which provides the CPT code and the timing code. The receptionist will give this to the patient to look over and sign. The patient will have to keep one copy for his or her own records. The patient can review when the doctor receives payment. This is for auditing purposes only, in case there is a necessity to do an audit in the future. Currently, the electronic medical record with practice management can perform the above function.

NHCS should set up two procedure codes, one for evaluation and management (E&M) and one for a time code. E&M is a doctor taking the patient's history, performing the examination, making a diagnosis, and treating the patient. Some medical specialties may use the E&M code, but some specialties may use the time code. For example, a pediatrician might spend a significant amount of time with a child, but his or her E&M may be low, so the practitioner can use the time code instead of E&M. On the other hand, an endocrinologist's E&M might be high, but the time spent with the patient may be short, so the practitioner can bill with the E&M.

The time code is an objective measure, and the E&M code is more subjective. The time code is a better fee-pay-ment schedule in a doctor's office if every one agrees that time is money. For example, if one doctor can do E&M in a shorter amount of time because he or she is very sharp and up-to-date on the latest medical knowledge, then he or she can see more patients. Another doctor can see the same patient with the same disease, but he or she might take a longer time to do E&M; he or she might get more payment because he or she takes a longer amount of time, but he or she cannot see as many patients as the smarter doctor. Therefore, NHCS should set a fee schedule for the time code. Payment for the first half hour should be 100 percent; the next additional fifteen minutes will pay at 75 percent; the next additional fifteen minutes will pay at 50 percent, and so on. Since the first half hour pays 100 percent of the fee, it will encourage the doctor to update his or her medical knowledge and improve his or her E&M skills so he or she can see more patients at 100 percent payment.

Payment Upper Limit Setup

The health care business originates from the basic units, the patient and the doctor. This is a very private business deal. It is very difficult and cumbersome for any outside agency to handle this business. After twenty-nine years in private practice, experience tells me that the best way to handle this business is to let honest doctors have their own autonomy and let them do what they think is best for their patients.

If a provider generates a significant income, it should trigger auditing. Each specialty's consensus committee (appointed by NHCS) should set an upper limit for income. The NHCS will set up the policy, if necessary, for auditing those doctors who reach or exceed the upper limit for payment in each specialty. This is similar to the U.S. IRS system. If it is necessary, the IRS will audit people with an income beyond a certain level; for example, over two hundred thousand dollars per year for a family practitioner. This payment upper limit should be adjusted every year or two. This upper limit will prevent bad providers from cheating or stealing taxpayers' money by making fraudulent claims and prevent one doctor from seeing too many patients and creating medical error. This policy should be included inside the contract.

NHCS will set up a Web site for doctors to check their income payment. When the practitioners reach the upper limit payment, practitioners must choose between the following:

(1). They can continue as usual, but they may get audited. As long as they keep their records straight and they are honest, they should not be afraid of auditing.

(2). They can slow down their practice, taking more time for their family or a personal hobby.

(3). They can see patients free of charge. This is for pursuing self-satisfaction and happiness.

Another problem that this upper limit addresses is the problem of one doctor seeing too many patients. Recently, ABC News gave a report on a doctor who operated on the wrong site on the body (2007). If one doctor sees too many patients, he or she may forget which site to operate upon because the doctor did not have time to review the case and he or she is very tired. The case may have been scheduled a few weeks ago, and the surgeon cannot remember because he or she is so busy.

In the United States, it is the hospital operating room set-up policy that, in all cases, before an operation starts, the nurse will announce a time-out to check the patient's ID, which site is to be operated on, and what kind of surgery is to be performed. Nevertheless, even with those precautions, mistakes are sometimes made.

Preauthorization

There should be two forms for preauthorization: a general form and a special form. The general form tries to prevent overutilization of treatment or surgical procedures. NHCS should consult with the college of each medical specialty and outline the indications and criteria for types of diagnoses and treatments based on the feedback from each college. The information would be contained within a form as a reminder to assist doctors with their decisions. The practitioner fills out the form and does the self-preauthorization and stores this in the electronic medical record. This policy will avoid the huge administrative costs of doing preauthorizations.

The practitioner should then print out two copies. One copy is given to the patient and the practitioner should explain to the patient why surgery or special treatment is necessary. One copy is put into the practitioner's chart for the record. This is only for future auditing purposes, if it becomes necessary.

The special form requires written or, if urgent, phone-call authorization. I estimate that about 5 to 10 percent of procedures or special treatments need to have a written request or call for urgent authorization. There are three ways to handle this issue:

(1). By a special and rare case-by-case procedure—The NHCS director should get the consensus from each college of medical specialty on which procedures require fax or telephone-call authorization.

(2). By price tag—If the procedure or treatment costs more than, for example, ten thousand dollars, then it needs special preauthorization.

(3). By combining the above two ways.

Consumers are concerned about freedom of treatment or a long wait for treatment. NHCS will let the doctor do what is best for his or her patient. Under the doctor's contract, there is a policy for authorization for treatment. Doctors use self-authorization; therefore, a patient cannot complain to NHCS. In order to prevent overutilization of self-authorization, NHCS will monitor doctors' behavior. This will ensure that a doctor does the right thing for his or her patient. A doctor's behavior will be monitored in the following two ways: First, when a doctor's income reaches the upper limit, the computer monitoring this will show a yellow alert. If the doctor's income is going to go over a certain level, the computer will transmit the information to the doctor's college of specialty for review (NHCS will contract with each college of specialty to do the review). If the review board finds that a doctor is guilty of any wrongdoing, then NHCS will terminate that doctor's contract and send a report to the state medical board for review. Second, if there are too many self-authorizations (NHCS will decide how many is too many) or serious complications after treatment, then the computer will transmit the information to the doctor's college of specialty for review. The review board will report back to NHCS, which will take the recommended actions.

Malpractice Issue

Each provider should have an arbitration agreement with each patient. NHCS will post the arbitration-agreement contract on its Web site. NHCS should also contract with several insurance companies to sell low-cost malpractice insurance to the providers. If a patient does not want to sign an arbitration agreement and the provider wants to see this patient, then the provider has to buy his or her own separate private insurance to cover malpractice for those who do not want to sign the arbitration agreement.

Medical Court

NHCS needs to establish a medical court. This medical court should be separate from other civil courts. This special court is just for medical-practice liability. This will save billions of dollars in medical costs because a health care provider will not order or perform unnecessary tests or procedures to prevent a medical-malpractice suit from taking place in civil court. The medical court should consist of a specially trained judge with medical knowledge and an evidence base as a guideline. The economic (actual medical costs for treatment) and noneconomic (pain and suffering) damages should be paid according to a schedule of compensation for each specific type of injury.

The plaintiff and the defense attorney should submit their documents, and the judge will decide who is right and conclude the case within three months. Then the judge will award the amount of damages according the compensation schedule, which should be established by a committee. The judge also will assign what percentage should be paid to the winning attorney. If the defeated attorney does not agree with the judge, he or she can appeal the case. The appeal will be assigned to three out-of-state judges, and the name of the original judge will be concealed. If the three appellate judges decide that the original judge made a serious deviation from standard judgment, then the three appellate judges can fire the original judge, and the three judges can fine the original judge severely. If the three judges agree with the original judge, the case will be closed.

6

Hospital Contract

This is an important sector for NHCS to control the cost of health care.

Ideally, NHCS should set up the guidelines for every state and every county, including the ideal number of hospitals and how many beds each county will need. The only exception is in rural areas, where NHCS should form a special task force to investigate each particular rural area and come up with the number of hospitals it needs. It is similar to the city plan. Every city needs to design a plan of its own.

Basic Requirement

NHCS will sign a contract with the hospital that passes the basic performance score.

Performance Score Setup

NHCS will set up a points-based scoring system for hospital performance. The scoring system consists of a Joint Commission on Accreditation of Healthcare Organizations (JCAHO) report, or NHCS can create a performance scoring system; a consumers' feedback report, and a providers' feedback report;

Since advanced information technology is available now, NHCS can collect performance scores easily; for example, a hospital's surgical complication rate (how often complications happen with particular surgical procedure). NHCS should design a special CPT code for complication cases in that particular surgical procedure. When a hospital bills for this complication code, the computer will put this into the hospital's profile database automatically. If the hospital wants to cheat and does not bill for this complication code, then NHCS can audit the cases if necessary or set up a toll-free telephone number for patients to call in.

NHCS will put all those reports together and assign points to each hospital. All hospital performance scores should be available to all citizens via Web site, newspaper, or postal mail. Hospitals should be allowed to compete using their performance scores in order to attract more patients.

Hospital CEO Qualifications

NHCS will require that hospital administrators or CEOs be medical doctors. Hospital CFOs should be business administrators. Currently, about 4 percent of U.S. hospital administrators are medical doctors.

A hospital takes care of medical business. If a medical doctor is in charge of hospital operations, he or she should operate the hospital in a more efficient way in regard to a value-based result (Porter 2006). He or she will not only contain costs and control waste, but also achieve the highest quality of medical care possible. He or she will coordinate with the medical staff to achieve this.

Ideally, special units in the hospital should have a medical director in charge, especially in units with high operating costs, such as the operating rooms, labor and delivery (L&D) rooms, and the ICU. Each medical specialty should elect members to form a committee and oversee patients' care. They will report outcome of care to the hospital administrator and to all medical staff. Those members involved in the hospital's quality-of-care committee must get appropriate compensation in order to perform their job seriously. The members can rotate every year. This is a very important issue concerning hospital operation.

Patients in the hospital belong to the doctors (they are the doctors' patients), not the hospital, so doctors have an obligation to check and monitor their patients' safety and the quality of care in the hospital. It is a direct measurement of health care performance, as opposed to outsiders, who simply look for the data collected and compiled by hospital personnel. However, it is very difficult for a doctor to carry out this process because doctors are busy, and some are not interested in hospital operation.

A nurse's medical knowledge is not always equal to that of a doctor. For example, in a labor and delivery room, hospitals let the unit's nursing director design the protocol for admitting a patient. I have seen one hospital labor and delivery form; there are about twenty to forty pages for the labor and delivery nurse to fill out. There are many unnecessary questions, and there is much duplicated information. That information is in the doctor's prenatal record. If one nurse has to spend so much time filling out the form, then that nurse does not have enough time to take care of a patient. There are two options: (a) the hospital hires more nurses and increases the hospital's operating cost, or (b) the hospital pays less to the nurse. If reimbursement rates are fixed, a hospital will operate in the red. A hospital administrator (whose major is in business only) cannot figure out why that unit loses money even though the nursing director is working very hard and the nurses are doing a good job. A medical director can step in and easily figure out the root causes.

Hospital Government Board

Government board members should consist of 50 percent hospital medical staff members and 50 percent local community representatives. This is for balance of voting power.

Payment Schedule

Fee payment should be based on the basic national rate and the hospital's performance score.

Bundle CPT Code

Hospital inpatient services should use a bundle CPT code for the following services:

(1) Pathologist—for the department of laboratory medicine.

(2) Radiologist—for the department of imaging services.

(3) Anesthesiologist—for the department of anesthesiology.

These services need to have a bundle CPT code. For example, currently in the United States, fees paid to an anesthesiologist are determined by time card; the longer a patient stays in the operating room, the more payment the anesthesiologist gets. This sounds reasonable, but unfortunately, it is a mistake. An anesthesiologist may be in the operating room the entire time. If she or he is paid according to the amount of time she or he spends in the room, she or he has no motivation to ensure that procedures are not prolonged. Pathologists and radiologists, on the other hand, never see the patient. When they bill the patient, the patient may not know who those doctors are and why the charges are so high.

The above three entities of medical services should bundle their fees together (the professional's fee and facility's fee) because an insurance company has a limited budget; if an insurance company pays the hospital and the doctor separately, the hospital always requests an increase in the reimbursements fee every year when it submits expenditures data to the insurance company. The insurance company has to pay more to the hospital because the hospital has expenses data to support its claims, but doctors do not have any data to support their charges. Their professional worth is very difficult to quantify. Therefore, the insurance company must decrease payment to the doctor to contain costs. If a doctor does not agree, the insurance company will contract with another doctor because there are plenty of doctors who will be willing to take less. This is unfair to the doctor; most doctors do not know this strategy. In the United States, practicing doctors have received less fee reimbursement every year for the past five to ten years (Lipthrott 2004).

When NHCS signs a contract with a hospital, NHCS policy must state that payment to radiologists, pathologists, and anesthesiologists in a hospital will include both the practitioner's professional fee and the facility fee. NHCS policy also needs to spell out how the total amount should be allocated, for example, 30 percent to the radiologist and 70 percent to the hospital facility per case. NHCS should hire people to figure out the appropriate ratio, then NHCS should decide the ratio and adjust it yearly.

NHCS should prohibit a hospital from paying a fixed salary to a radiologist, pathologist, or anesthesiologist. If the hospital pays a fixed salary to a practitioner, the hospital will find the practitioners who are willing to get less payment and disregard the practitioners' quality.

7

Outpatient Laboratory Service Contract

Performance Score Setup

NHCS will set up the criteria for standard performance and will sign a contract with those laboratories that pass the standard performance requirements.

NHCS should schedule inspections regularly, or require that laboratories self-report via the Internet.

Laboratory Request Form

NHCS will design a software program for ordering laboratory tests. When a doctor orders a test, he or she must fill out the request form via Web site, then send it to the laboratory by fax, e-mail, or printout and give a copy of it to the patient. The request form should be designed by an NHCS expert (NHCS will consult with the laboratory director and the doctor). The request forms should contain a questionnaire. The ordering doctor must answer why he or she is ordering the test (what indications there are), plus a tentative diagnosis code. All those procedures must be carried out by the software program, which will be available in the doctor's office. This will reduce many unnecessary tests because there will be a record in each doctor's data profile. NHCS can monitor each practitioner's ordering behavior.

NHCS should supply the software program to each laboratory facility and provider. This uniform system will save huge medical costs because many practitioners order unnecessary tests without restrictions.

8

Outpatient Imaging Service Contract

Performance Score Setup

NHCS will set up the criteria for outpatient imaging center performance standard requirements.

Fee Schedule

NHCS will set up a fee schedule. Ideally, one procedure code should include professional services and the facility. (The facility may be owned by a doctor, a business corporation, or a hospital.) This is a bundle fee. It should not make a difference who owns the facility. NHCS will spell out the percentage of payment that goes to the radiologist and to the facility. NHCS will consult experts who will figure out the reasonable fees for the doctor and for the facility.

Request Form

There are two components to monitoring the ordering of tests. NHCS should design the software for ordering tests (NHCS should consult a radiologist), and NHCS should set a cap on payment per procedure per month.

When a doctor orders a test, the ordering doctor must fill out the request form using NHCS software. The request form should ask why the doctor is ordering the test (what is the indication) and what the tentative diagnosis code is. Subsequent interactive questions will follow in order to avoid unnecessary tests. Please refer to the section on monitoring practitioner behavior in chapter five for a detailed explanation.

The calculation of the upper limit for payment will be based on the facility's equipment costs, capital expenditure, and mortgage payment monthly as well as the radiologist's average monthly salary. If the imaging center reaches the maximum payment, it cannot receive any more payment. The radiologist then has the following two choices: First, any additional order will be free of charge as a charity donation. Second, the radiologist should ask the ordering doctor why the test was ordered. This will make the ordering doctor more cautious.

It is my estimation that many tests are unnecessary because the ordering doctor does not know the indications for the test and may not know the limitations of the information one can get from that test. There is not adequate special education or training regarding this for doctors during their years in medical school or in their postgraduate residency training, especially for modern, more expensive technology.

9

Special Medical Clinic Contract

Special Medical Clinic

The special medical clinic is a total health care delivery clinic. The clinic is for chronic diseases only: diabetes, stroke (recovery from acute stage), chronic mental disorder (dementia, Alzheimer's disease, etc.), chronic heart disease (congestive heart failure, coronary heart disease, chronic hypertension), chronic pulmonary diseases, cancer (medical treatment after surgery and radiation), chronic kidney disease (dialysis), rheumatologic disease, HIV, and "bad lifestyle" diseases (alcoholism, smoking, and obesity).

Program Setup

The clinic program should include: patient education, medical treatment, rehabilitation, follow-up and monitoring, and collection and reporting of the patient's medical-treatment outcome.

Fee Schedule

NHCS will set up the reimbursement rate according to the performance of the clinic. Contract reimbursement rates will vary in each clinic. This will create competition among clinics to demonstrate better health care outcomes. The special medical clinic is the ideal health care sector in which to apply the HMO model. Because this is a chronic-disease treatment center, NHCS should pay the clinic as a total health care entity instead of paying by fee-for-service.

10

Specialized Surgical Center Contract

The specialized surgical center is the health care center that can create the best value-based health care outcome (Porter 2006). It will be a center of excellence. The center should be well organized and well equipped with up-to-date technology. Surgeons should have both good medical knowledge and good surgical skills. The facility can be inside an existing hospital, but it should operate under a separate unit, or it can be an independent surgical center. This is for monitoring quality of care results and for reimbursement rate calculation.

Specialized Surgical Center

The following categories belong to the specialized surgical center:

(1). Orthopedic surgery

(2). Thoracic (open-heart and pulmonary) surgery

(3). Neurosurgery

(4). Cancer surgery

Criteria for Specialized Surgical Center Setup

The center should set up the minimum number of each procedure to be performed in a month. Doctors should have specialty board certification. The center should set up a required minimum number of each procedure performed by each doctor. The center needs to have a medical director in charge of all operations. He or she also is responsible for collecting all data of patients' care outcomes.

In my intensive observation over thirty years, I have seen that the best surgical outcome depends on the surgeon's good medical knowledge and excellent surgical skill in a well-organized surgical team. Expensive surgical instruments or equipment are needed only for a few special surgical procedures.

Obstetric Delivery Center

In order to set up the center, a board-certified obstetrician must be in the facility twenty-four hours a day and seven days a week; a board-certified perinatologist should be available for consultation twenty-four hours a day and seven days a week; a board-certified neonatologist must be in the facility twenty-four hours a day and seven days a week; a board-certified midwife could do routine deliveries in the center under an obstetrician's supervision; and a medical director should be in charge of the center's operation. The medical director will collect the patient's care outcomes and reports. A center can be located inside an existing hospital but as a separate operating unit, or it can be an independent delivery center, equipped with a C-section and a life-saving emergency operation setup. This independent center (not in the hospital) should only accept normal pregnancy patients, and no high-risk pregnancies.

The center (if not inside a hospital setting) should have a transport ambulance and be able to transfer patients or newborns to a hospital for further care after the patient's or newborn's condition is stable.

This obstetric delivery center will cost less to operate, and will result in a higher quality of care. It will reduce many obstetric malpractice suits if all the criteria are met.

11

Health Care Outcome

Data Collection

A performance report for individual practitioners and a value-based data report (Potter 2006) from hospital, special clinics, laboratories, imaging centers, and medical device companies should be created. NHCS can hire people inside the department to collect the data on health care quality and care outcomes or it may contract with companies that have had many years of experience in data collection.

Report on Health Care Outcomes

The director of NHCS will use this report to amend the policy and improve the performance of all health care providers. NHCS will publish performance scores on its Web site. Citizens will then be able to make wiser choices when selecting their care providers.

12

Accessory Health Care

The following three entities belong to the category of accessory health care: prescription drugs, dental care, and long-term care.

For its accessory health care policy, NHCS should set up the regulations for private insurances to sell these accessory health care plans. This is because accessory health care is a direct contract between patients and insurance companies, and whether a citizen needs these is dependent on his or her individual circumstances. However, most citizens can afford to pay an insurance plan's premium. Those citizens whose incomes are below poverty level, according the state's definition, can get help from the state or county to sponsor a plan for free or a minimal charge.

Prescription Drugs

NHCS will pay for hospital, outpatient and ambulatory surgical center, or institution drug treatment. If a patient returns to the doctor's office for short-term prescription drug medications, the patient must pay for the prescription drug costs.

Why should the patient pay for office-prescribed drugs? This is to avoid patients' abuse of the system or the overutilization of drugs. Most patients can afford to pay for short-term prescription drugs. If a citizen's income is below the state's poverty level, he or she can apply for a state-sponsored prescription drug program. If a patient knows that he or she has to take drugs for a long time, he or she should apply for a private insurance–sponsored prescription drug plan or an NHCS-sponsored prescription drug plan.

Patents for new drugs should be under a special subdivision of the patent office. This subdivision of the patent office should be under the Food and Drug Administration's (FDA) control. Drug patents should be separate from all other patents; they should not belong to the regular patent office.

Drug companies spend huge sums of money to do research (especially for biopharmaceutical drugs), therefore they want to get their money back for those expenses. I agree that they should be reimbursed. However, how long will it take for those companies to get their money back?

Here, the FDA should step in. A division of the FDA that specializes in drug pricing should grant a patent to the drug company. The patent could allow the drug company to sell the drug either at a higher price for a fewer number of years or for a lower price for a longer period of time. This would allow the drug company to get back its investment. Like a mortgage payment, each month's payment should be less for a five-year loan than for a three-year loan. If the new drug is very expensive to make, the FDA should give this new drug a longer patent so the drug company can sell the drug at a lower price.

Remember, the goal of curing human diseases is not indulging in material, luxury things. Drug companies should not make a huge profit on human suffering.

Dental Care

Each state should provide dental care to those citizens whose income falls below state poverty level. The state should issue a dental care card free of charge or for a minimal charge.

Long-Term Care

Long-term care includes a variety of services that apply to people with a chronic illness or a disability. The majority of people who require long-term care are senior citizens or disabled people. Services include medical and nonmedical care.

Citizens should take care of their own long-term care. Long-term care greatly depends upon each individual's needs. NHCS should adopt the U.S. Medicare program's policy regarding long-term care. It is a fair policy; generally, Medicare doesn't pay for long-term care. Medicare pays only for a medically necessary skilled nursing facility or medically necessary home health care. However, you must meet certain conditions for Medicare to pay for these types of care. Most long-term care includes support services for activities of daily living, such as dressing, bathing, and using the bathroom. Medicare doesn't pay for this type of care, which is called "custodial care"(non-skilled care). For older people with low incomes and limited assets, a state or federal government program can pay for certain health services, such as a nursing home, or care at home and in the community.

Conclusion

The United States of America should reform its health care system right now. It is estimated that about forty to fifty million people have no health insurance. Those legal residents have no insurance either because the insurance premium is too high, and they cannot afford to pay; or because they assume that the insurance premium is low, but they think it is unnecessary to buy health insurance because they are healthy.

Currently, most politicians are proposing universal health care—a multi-payer system by the Democratic Party, and a free-market system by the Republican Party. Both systems are doomed to failure. There is no way the congress can pass or enforce a law requiring private insurance carriers to sell low-cost or affordable health insurance plans. If private insurance carriers cannot make money, they will close their operation. Politicians are just focused on uninsured citizens' problems, but privately insured citizens also have serious problems with very high insurance premiums. Under a single-payer system, the government health care tax would be much less than private insurance companies' insurance premiums. According to my estimation, consumers will pay about one third of the cost of a private insurance premium. This estimation is based on the fact that private insurance companies spend about one third of the premiums for administration and one third for profits. Another serious problem of universal health care (in multi-payer mode) is that it creates multiple managers; not only will this create high administrative costs, but it will also create inefficiency and disorganized health care system management. Right now in the United States, the key problems are in the management of the health care system. In my personal experience, the health care efficiency of current private insurance companies in the United States is worse than the public single-payer system (Medicare). For example, I called a private insurance carrier regarding a patient's claim issues, and it took a long time for their employee (overseas) to answer the issues I raised, and they still have not been completely resolved. When I had the same problem with another patient, I called Medicare, spoke to an employee there, and the employee resolved the issue very quickly.

My plans are as follows:

(1). Uninsured citizens or citizens who do not pay income tax need to purchase a low-cost health plan from NHCS (in my suggested single-payer system, the fee charged will be the same as or less than the general taxation, depending on the patient's age and for how long the card is effective), or a plan from a private insurance company. This policy needs to be enforced by documentation when a citizen applies for or renews his or her driver's license. For those citizens who are below the state poverty level, the state must pay into the general tax for them. Every year, those citizens who live below poverty level need to apply for renewal. The state also has an obligation to publish their names on a Web site, so that all state citizens know who is receiving state help to pay for their health care. The citizens who get help from their fellow citizens must work harder and take care of their personal health issues more carefully. After all, no one can help thee forever except thyself. I emphasize this point in my book *An Intimate Relationship: Genes, Cancer, Lifestyle, and You* (2007).

(2). Get the support of many large corporations who need to pay very high medical insurance premiums for their employees. The larger corporations will establish a higher profit margin by using this system, and they will be able to prevent jobs from moving overseas to avoid the high insurance premium for a domestic employee. The government will therefore gain more income-tax revenue.

(3). Set up the Department of the National Health Care System and search for an NHCS director to organize the department.

(4). During this transitional period, NHCS can adopt the model of the Medicare system administered by CMS (Center for Medicare and Medicaid Services), their personnel, and their technologies.

(5). Regarding the existing Medicare program, there are two options. The department can continue the program until Medicare fund contributions end but put CMS under NHCS supervision in order to simplify the system and save huge administrative fees. Alternatively, the department can merge the Medicare program with NHCS, and those senior citizens who contribute funds to the program would not need to pay the health care general tax.

(6). An NHCS health care budget of about 10 percent of the GDP (compared to current total health care expenditures of about 16 to 17 percent of the GDP in the United States) will be enough to cover all citizens, in my estimation. If NHCS follows the suggestions in this book to contain costs, it most likely may spend less than 10 percent of the GDP. There is no middleman fee. Instead, most health care money goes to consumers and providers. This would be comparable to health care expenditures in Switzerland, Germany, Canada, and France. If my theory is correct, and a single-payer system can save one third of the current spending by reducing administrative costs and one third of the current spending, which goes toward profits for private insurance, then the NHCS health care budget will be comparable to health care expenditures in the United Kingdom, about 7 to 8 percent of the GDP (OECD 2006).

If the candidate who becomes president of the United States of America in 2008 can carry out universal health care with the single-payer system that I outline here, I can predict that he or she will be remembered as a great president.

Health care is very complex. While there is no one person who can address the entire picture, this book addresses some ways in which current problems can be addressed. If the health care system proposed is created, it will continue to be refined over the years. The system is based around the relationship between the doctor and patient. However, many specialties and agencies would also play a part under the NHCS umbrella in order to address all needs. I emphasize that no second parties should be involved in financial management between providers and consumers. The policy I recommend would provide for doctor oversight and patient education. It would provide quality care at an affordable price.

The following story is one example of how a doctor receives great rewards from practicing medicine. I received a letter and picture from my patient recently, and he invited me to attend his graduation from California Polytechnic. I delivered this boy by C-section twenty-four years ago. He had gastroschisis (a congenital abdominal defect, the intestine is outside the abdomen). The mother was very young, and we were very scared at that time because it is a very rare congenital anomaly. He was a very skinny boy when he was five months old. Now he is six feet and two inches tall and one hundred sixty-five pounds, and he looks very handsome. I was so thrilled that my tears were dripping when I got the letter and his picture. This is the true reward in my medical practice career.

References

8th Annual Tamkin Symposium. 2006. *Health Care for All: Is the Dream Possible?* University of California, Irvine School of Medicine, Irvine, California. October 31, 2006.

ABC News 2007. "Surgical Mishaps: Wrong-Site Operations." August 9, 2007. http://abcnews.go.com/GMA/OnCall/story?id=3459845&page=1.

Abelson, Julia, et al. 2004. "Canadians Confront Health Care Reform." *Health Affairs* 23, no. 3 (May/June): 186–193.

Amelung, Volker, Sherry Glied, and Angelina Topan. 2003. "Health Care and the Labor Market: Learning from the German Experience." *Journal of Health Politics, Policy and Law* 28, no. 4:695–714.

Andersen, Ronald, Bjorn Smedby, and Denny Vagero. 2001. "Cost Containment, Solidarity and Cautious Experimentation: Swedish Dilemmas." *Social Science & Medicine* 52 (2001): 1195–1204.

BarackObama.com. "Creating a Healthcare System that Works." www.barackobama.com

Chen, Charles H., MD, FACOG. *An Intimate Relationship: Genes, Cancer, Lifestyle, and You.* Lincoln, Nebraska: iUniverse, 2007.

Cheng, Tsung-Mei. 2003. "Taiwan's New National Health Insurance Program: Genesis and Experience So Far." *Health Affairs* 22, no. 3 (May/June): 61–76.

Cranovsky, Richard, et al. 2000. "Health Technology Assessment in Switzerland." *International Journal of Technology Assessment in Health Care* 16 no. 2 (2000): 576–590.

Davis, Karen, et al. "Slowing the Growth of U.S. Health Care Expenditures: What are the Options?" *The Commonwealth Fund/Alliance for Health Reform.* Bipartisan Congressional Health Policy Conference, 2007.

Day, Patricia, and Rudolf Klein. 1991. "Britain's Health Care Experiment." *Health Affairs* (Fall): 39–59.

Defino, Theresa. 2006. "Critical Condition: Three Big Ideas for Saving Our Ailing Healthcare System." *Physicians Practice* (February): 33–40.

Gutierrez, Susana M. Borroto, Tsutomu Mizota, and Yasuyuki Rakue. 2003. "Comparison of Four Health Systems: Cuba, China, Japan and the U.S.A., an Approach to Reality." *Southeast Asian Journal Tropical Medicine Public Health* 34, no. 4 (December):

Health Affairs: The Policy Journal of the Health Sphere. www.healthaffairs.org

HillaryClinton.com. "American Health Choices Plan." www.hillaryclinton.com

Hurst, Jeremy M. 1991. "Reforming Health Care in Seven European Nations." *Health Affairs* (Fall): 7–21.

Hussey, P. and G. F. Anderson. 2003. "A Comparison of Single-and Multi-Payer Health Insurance Systems and Options for Reform." *Health Policy* 66, 215–228.

Ikegami, Naoki, and John Creighton Campbell. 2004. "Japan's Health Care System: Containing Costs and Attempting Reform." *Health Affairs* 23, no. 3 (May/ June): 26–36.

Inquiry: The Journal of Health Care Organization, Provision, and Financing. www.inquiryjournal.org.

John Edwards for President. "Universal Health Care through Shared Responsibility." www.johnedwards.com.

Journal of Healthcare Management. www.ache.org.

Lipthrott, Dawn. 2004. *Ethical Health Partnerships.* www.ethicalhealthpartnerships.org.

Lu, Jui-Fen Rachel, and William C. Hsiao. 2003. "Does Universal Health Insurance Make Health Care Unaffordable? Lessons from Taiwan." *Health Affairs* 22, no. 3 (2003): 77–88.

McCormick, Danny, MD, David U. Himmelstein, MD, and David H. Bor, MD. 2004. "Single-Payer National Health Insurance." *Archives of Internal Medicine* 164 (February): 300–304.

McGlynn, Elizabeth A. 2004. "There Is No Perfect Health System." *Health Affairs* 23, no. 3 (May/June): 100–102.

Mello, Michelle M., David M. Studdert, and Troyen A. Brennan. 2003. "The Leapfrog Standards: Ready to Jump from Marketplace to Courtroom?" *Health Affairs* 22, no. 2: 46–59.

OECD (Organization for Economic Cooperation and Development) Health Data 2002. Paris: OECD, 2002; and R. J. Lu and W. C. Hsiao, "Development of Taiwan's National Health Account," *Taiwan Economic Review* 29, no. 4 (2001).

OECD (Organization for Economic Cooperation and Development) Health Data 2006. www.oecd.org/health/healthdata.

Porter, Michael E., and Elizabeth Olmsted Teisberg. *Redefining Health Care: Creating Value-Based Competition on Results.* Boston, MA: Harvard Business School Press, 2006.

Reinhardt, Uwe E., Peter S. Hussey, and Gerard F. Anderson. 2004. "U.S. Health Care Spending in an International Context." *Health Affairs* 23, no. 3: 10–25.

Rosen, Per, and Ingvar Karlberg. 2002. "Opinions of Swedish Citizens, Health-Care Politicians, Administrators and Doctors on Rationing and Health-Care Financing." *Health Expectation* 5: 148–155.

Schut, Frederik T., Stefan Greb, and Juergen Wasem. 2003. "Consumer Price Sensitivity and Social Health

Insurer Choice in Germany and the Netherlands." *International Journal of Health Care Finance and Economics* 3: 117–138.

Smith, Peter C., and Nick York. 2004. "Quality Incentives: The Case of U.K. General Practitioners." *Health Affairs* 23, no. 3 (May/June): 112–118.

Stevens, Simon. 2004. "Reform Strategies for the English NHS." *Health Affairs* 23, no. 3 (May/June): 37–44.

Urban Institute. "Medicare Outperforms Private Insurance at Containing Health Care Spending, and on Several Measures." March 11, 2003. www.urban.org.

Zynx Health. www.zynx.com.

Index

978-0-595-47158-4
0-595-47158-7